THYROID HEALING

DIET RECIPES

COOKBOOK:

50 New Research-Based Recipes To Help Free The Body From Hashimoto's, Graves', Hypothyroidism & Thyroid Related Problems

Copyright Page

All rights reserved. No part of this publication may be reproduced, distributed, or transmitted in any form or by any means, including photocopying, recording, or other electronic or mechanical methods, without the prior written permission of the publisher, except in the case of brief quotations embodied in critical reviews and certain other noncommercial uses permitted by copyright law.

Copyright © 2017

BRIAN MED

Table of Contents

INTRODUCTION 5

What Is Hypothyroidism? 6

An Overview on Hashimoto's thyroiditis 7

Causes Of Hashimoto's Thyroiditis?... 8

Who Is At Risk?... 9

Early Signs & Symptoms Of Hashimoto's Thyroiditis.................................. 10

New Recipes To Rescue The Thyroid.. 11

Creamy Lime Pudding 11

Baked Stuffed Pumpkin 12

Thyroid Diet Oyster Pancake... 13

Amaranth Porridge.. 15

Berry Clafoutis... 16

Ginger & Strawberry Cobbler.. 17

Chicory Latte 18

Almond Zucchini Apple Pancakes 19

Veggie Roast & Moroccan Spice 20

Fish Ferment 21

Stir Fry Mushroom Leek 22

Lamb Sausages with Cucumbers... 23

Tahini & Mustard Chicken Spread 24

Chia Seed Pudding 25

R. Sweet Potato Wedges... 26

Braised Green Cabbage.. 27

Arugula Smoked Fish... 28

Veggie & Sausage Delight 29

Fish Soup 30

Coconut Almond Banana Muffins 31

Salad Recipes... 32

Zucchini & Anchovy Salad 32

Raw Beetroot & Orange Salad 33

Tahini Miso Dressing 34

3

Prebiotic Creamy Potato Salad 35

Creamy Broccoli Salad... 36

Seaweed Cucumber Salad.. 37

Steamed Collard Greens 38

Sauerkraut Cumin Salad 39

Roasted B. Tomatoes Over Kale... 40

Arugula & Baby Tomatoes Mix 41

Smoothies & Tea **42**

Eggless Mayonnaise 42

Avocado & Cocoa Smoothie... 43

Super Boost Green Basil Smoothie 44

Pumpkin Smoothie... 45

Goji Grapefruit Smoothie... 46

Blackberry Power Smoothie... 47

Improved Homemade Ginger Ale 48

Root C. Green Smoothie 49

Root C. Green Smoothie 2 50

Thyroid Power Smoothie 51

Berry Green Smoothie 52

Thyroid Green Smoothie.. 53

Thyroid Booster Smoothie... 54

Green Tea Smoothie 55

Mango Inspired Smoothie.. 56

Blueberry Choco Delight 57

Pina Colada Smoothie 58

Homemade Cola drink 59

Dairy-Free Turmeric Chai Latte 60

Lemon Ginger Tea 61

Conclusion **62**

INTRODUCTION

Congratulations and thank you for downloading this book: *THYROID HEALING DIET RECIPES COOKBOOK: 50 New Research-Based Recipes To Help Free The Body From Hashimoto's, Graves', Hypothyroidism & Thyroid Related Problems.*

Contained herein, are the 50 new research-based recipes proven to be effective, in helping you combat Hashimoto's thyroiditis and heal your thyroid forever.

The recipes are gluten-free, dairy-free and also, healthy and delicious. They contain a lot of proven steps and the truth behind Hashimoto's thyroiditis. These recipes will give you real hope and help you discover real reasons and the healing path for dozens of symptoms and conditions, including:

- aches and pains
- anxiety and depression
- autoimmune disease
- brain fog and focus
- cancer
- epstein-Barr virus
- pregnancy complications
- fatigue
- mononucleosis
- fibromyalgia and CFS
- hair thinning and loss
- hashimoto's thyroiditis
- headaches and migraines
- heart palpitations
- vertigo
- hyperthyroidism
- hypothyroidism
- menopausal symptoms
- mystery weight gain
- sleep disorders
- tingles and numbness

What Is Hypothyroidism?

Hypothyroidism in simple terms is a condition in which the thyroid gland is underactive and doesn't properly produce or release thyroid hormones. On a norm, the thyroid gland releases many crucial hormones that travel through our bloodstream to reach the receptors found throughout the whole body. So, a disturbance as such, in the thyroid can cause widespread, noticeable health problems.

A Recent study has it that 12 percent of Americans are likely to develop a thyroid condition at some point in their lives. While some estimates, suggests that up to 40 percent of the population suffers from at least some level of underactive thyroid.

Over that years, research has shown that women — especially older women — are the most susceptible group for developing hypothyroidism.

An Overview on Hashimoto's thyroiditis

Hashimoto's is an autoimmune disorder. It makes the immune system produce antibodies that attack the body's tissues and, in that process, negatively affect the thyroid function.

Facts have it that about 90 percent of hypothyroid cases are due to Hashimoto's disease! In the vast majority of cases, hypothyroidism is actually not the problem of the thyroid itself, but a condition caused by excessive reactions of the entire immune system.

Causes Of Hashimoto's Thyroiditis?

Research has shown that the development of autoimmune disorders is multifactorial. "Genetics, nutrition, environmental impacts, stress, hormone levels, and immune factors are part of the puzzle.

What most doctors cannot tell for sure, is the underlying causes of Hashimoto's disease (and therefore hypothyroidism). However, the below factors, are the most common causes.

1. Autoimmune reactions to the disease: They can attack tissue throughout the body, including the thyroid gland
2. Slim bowel syndrome and normal gastrointestinal function problems.
3. Common allergies, inflammatory foods such as gluten and dairy products.
4. Other widely consumed foods that cause sensitivity and intolerance, including grains and many food supplements.
5. Emotional stress
6. Nutritional deficiencies

Who Is At Risk?

As already discussed in the beginning of this book, women — especially the older ones, are the most susceptible group for developing hypothyroidism. Although, there are several risk factors that can make it more likely that you'll develop Hashimoto's disease at some point in your lifetime. These include;

1. **Being a Woman:** Many women than men have the tendency of getting Hashimoto's disease, for reasons we are not yet sure about. One of the reasons why women may be more sensitive is that they are more affected by stress/anxiety, which can have a serious effect on female hormones. According to the New York Times article on thyroiditis, 10 times more women than men suffer from thyroid disorders.

2. **Middle Ages:** Most people with Hashimoto's disease are people aged between 20 to 60 years. The highest risk is among people over the age of 50, and researchers believe that the risk only increases with age. Many women at age 60 suffer from hypothyroidism to some extent, but older women often times, cannot be diagnosed with thyroid disorders because they imitate symptoms of menopause

3. **Autoimmune Disease History:** If a family member had a Hashimoto or Thyroid Disorder, or was treated with other autoimmune disorders in the past, they are more likely to develop the disorder itself

4. **Smoking cigarettes**

5. **After recent trauma or a very large amount of stress**: Stress contributes to hormonal imbalances, such as adrenal insufficiency, causes changes in thyroid hormone conversion T4 to T3 and weakened immune system of the body

6. **Pregnancy and Postpartum:** Pregnancy affects thyroid hormones in many ways, and it is possible that some women develop antibodies against their own thyroid during or after pregnancy (called autoimmune after birth)

Early Signs & Symptoms Of Hashimoto's Thyroiditis

Some of the most common signs and symptoms of Hashimoto's disease include:

1. Depression and anxiety
2. Weight gain
3. fatigue
4. infertility
5. Feeling cold, even when others do not.
6. Painful problems such as constipation and bloating
7. Pain in the muscles
8. Swollen face, eyes, and stomach
9. Stiffness and swelling of the joints.
10. Hair loss, changes in hair texture or hair thinning.
11. Coarse and cracked skin
12. Wheezing
13. Frequent urination and excessive thirst
14. Low sexual desire or sexual dysfunction.
15. Cold, infection or more frequent illness due to poor immune function
16. Changes in the menstrual cycle, including absent or irregular periods and problems with infertility.

New Recipes To Rescue The Thyroid

Creamy Lime Pudding

Prep time: 15 mins
Total time: 15 mins
Serves: 4-6

Ingredients

1.5 cups of organic cashews
1 cup water
¼ cup coconut butter (Artisana brand preferable)
zest of one lime (must be organic)
2 tsp lime juice
1 tsp vanilla extract
½ tsp rose water (optional)
A pinch of salt
6 drops of stevia (optional)
2 tsp rose petals (optional for decoration)

How You Make It

1. Simply combine all the ingredients in your blender and blend on high until the pudding reaches a smooth and silky consistency.

2. Next, you pour into a serving bowl and place in the fridge to chill for at least an hour after which you sprinkle with rose petals and serve.

Baked Stuffed Pumpkin

Prep time: 25 mins
Cook time: 1 hour
Total time: 1 hour 25 mins
Serves: 6-8

Ingredients

1 medium size pumpkin
2 cups brown rice (cooked)
1½ cups of cranberries
1 cup chicken stock
2 tbsp of flaxseed meal (ground flax seed)
1 cup pecans (chopped)
2 tsp of salt
2 stalks of sage (chopped)
2 tbsp olive oil

How You Make It

1. First, preheat your oven to 400F. After which you cut the top of the pumpkin off with a sharp knife.

2. Scoop out the seeds of the pumpkin and rub the outside pumpkin with some olive oil.

3. When done, make the stuffing by combining all the ingredients together in a bowl.

4. Now, stuff the pumpkin and cover it up with the pumpkin top from step one.

5. Place on a tray and bake for an hour.

6. This can be served as a main or as a side dish.

Thyroid Diet Oyster Pancake

Prep time: 5 mins
Cook time: 20 mins
Total time: 25 mins
Serves: 4

Ingredients

4 large eggs
8 oz. of fresh oysters
1 red or green pepper
1 large leek (sliced in rings)
1 stick celery (chopped)
1 handful of parsley (chopped)
1 sprig of fresh rosemary (chopped)
2 tbsp of fish sauce
1 tsp of sea salt
1 cup of rice flour
2 tbsp of lard, beef tallow, ghee or coconut oil
1 tsp baking powder (omit if you are following the Thyroid-GAPS diet)

How You Make It

1. First, roast the pepper directly over stove fire while turning every few minutes till it's well charred and the skin peels off easily.

2. Next, melt the fat in a large frying pan after which you saute the leeks and celery in it till soft and slightly browned.

3. Once that is achieved, chop the roasted pepper and add them.

4. Now, beat the eggs in a bowl and add the fish sauce, salt, oysters, parsley and rosemary to it.

5. After that, combine the rice flour and baking powder in another bowl and slowly stir in the egg bowl to make a smooth batter.

6. Add the batter to the veggies in the pan and give them a gentle stir before covering.

7. Cook over medium heat for 15-20 minutes or until the top is firm.

14

Amaranth Porridge

Prep time: 15 mins
Cook time: 30 mins
Total time: 45 mins
Serves: 2

Ingredients

1 cup of amaranth
4 cups of filtered water
1 tbsp ghee
½ tsp mustard seeds
½ tsp cumin
½ tsp sea salt
1 tsp dry turmeric
½ inch fresh ginger, julienned
½ tsp apple cider vinegar (ACV) or lemon
1 tbsp raw unsalted butter or ghee
a handful of raw pumpkin seeds

How You Make It

1. First, melt them in a heavy-bottom pan and add the cumin, ginger and mustard seeds when hot.

2. Once the mustard seeds starts popping, add the water, amaranth, and salt to it and bring to a boil.

3. Once that is achieved, reduce heat to low-medium and cook covered for 30 minutes or until creamy and thick.

4. After that, remove from heat and add butter (or ghee), ACV and turmeric.

5. Finally, sprinkle with pumpkin seeds and serve.

Berry Clafoutis

Prep time: 15 mins
Cook time: 25 mins
Total time: 40 mins
Serves: 12

Ingredients

1 to 2 cups of fresh or frozen berries
1 tbsp organic coconut oil
2 eggs
1 cup coconut milk (preferably Native Forest since it's BPA-free)
½ tsp vanilla extract
⅓ cup coconut nectar
3 tbsp coconut flour
½ tsp sea salt

How You Make It

1. First, preheat your oven to 400F.

2. Next, you spread some coconut oil at the base of a 9" pie dish.

3. After that, you put the berries in the baking dish from step two and put them in the oven for 6 to 10 mins for them to start "sweating."

4. Once that's achieved, combine all the remaining ingredients by first mixing the wet and dried separately after which you combine both by whisking to make a smooth batter.

5. When done, take out the dish from the oven and pour the batter over the fruit.

6. Finally, bake for 20 to 25 minutes, or until the middle is firm.

Ginger & Strawberry Cobbler

Prep time: 20 mins
Cook time: 40 mins
Total time: 1 hour
Serves: 4 to 6

Ingredients

Filling
1-pound strawberries
1 tbsp mint (chopped)
1 tsp vanilla powder or extract
2 tbsp lime juice and zest of one lime
1 tbsp ginger (grated)
2 tsp arrowroot (or tapioca starch)
pinch of salt

Topping
½ cup ghee or coconut oil (melted)
1 tbsp maple syrup
1 cup finely shredded coconut flakes
¼ cup arrowroot (or tapioca starch)
½ tsp vanilla powder
pinch of salt

How You Make It

1. Begin by preheating your oven to 350F after which you combine all the filling ingredients in a bowl and toss to evenly cover the strawberries.

2. Next, place the mixture in a cast iron skillet or baking dish.

3. Take out a separate bowl and combine all the topping ingredients in it. Use your hands to work the ghee oil into the paste until it turns into a crumble.

4. After that spread the crumble evenly on top of the strawberries and bake for 30 to 40 minutes.

Note: For low histamine, replace the strawberries with apples, pears or blueberries.

Chicory Latte

Prep time: 2 mins
Cook time: 12 mins
Total time: 14 mins
Serves: 2

Ingredients

1 tbsp roasted chicory root
2 cups of water
1 tbsp roasted dandelion root
2 tbsp ghee, coconut butter or butter (if tolerated)
2 pitted dates
(nut or powder) fresh nutmeg

How You Make It

1. First, place the chicory and dandelion root in a pot and cover with water.

2. Next, bring to a boil after which you reduce the heat and simmer for 2 minutes.

3. When done, remove from heat and let it steep for 10 minutes, then strain and transfer to your blender.

4. Add the ghee and dates to the blender and blend for 1 minute.

5. Grate some fresh nutmeg and enjoy.

Almond Zucchini Apple Pancakes

Prep time: 10 mins
Cook time: 10 mins
Total time: 20 mins
Serves: 6

Ingredients

1 small zucchini (grated)
1 small apple (grated)
1 cup almond flour
½ tsp baking powder (kindly omit if you are doing GAPS)
½ tsp sea salt
2-3 tbsp almond butter
3 sprigs of fresh thyme (chopped)
3 eggs
1 tbsp honey
2 tbsp of coconut oil

How You Make It

1. First, combine the apples, thyme, zucchini, honey and almond butter in a bowl and combine the flour, baking powder and salt in another bowl.

2. After that slightly beat the eggs and combine all the ingredients.

3. Heat the coconut oil over medium-high heat and fry the pancakes in it for about 5 minutes per side, without burning.

4. When done, serve with yogurt and fresh fruit.

Veggie Roast & Moroccan Spice

Prep time: 15 mins
Cook time: 45 mins
Total time: 1 hour
Serves: 4-6

Ingredients

Veggies of your choice (We made use of asparagus, parsnip, leeks, and carrots)
2 tbsp coconut oil (melted)
sea salt
Ras El Hanout (a Moroccan spice blend)

How You Make It

1. First, preheat your oven to 425F.

2. Next, toss the veggies with the oil, sea salt, and Moroccan blend.

3. When done, lay them out on parchment paper and bake for 45 minutes.

Fish Ferment

Ingredients

3- 4 very fresh large herrings or mackerel
1-2 tbsp of salt per liter of the brine
5-7 bay leaves
fresh dill or some dill seeds
1 small white onion (peeled & sliced)
1 tbsp of peppercorns
1 tsp of coriander seeds
1 cup of kefir whey
a suitable glass jar

How You Make It

1. First, skin the fish and remove the large bones after which you cut into bite-size pieces.

2. Mix the fish pieces in a glass jar with the peppercorns, onion, coriander seeds, bay leaves, and dill seeds or dill herb.

3. Next, dissolve 1 tbsp of sea salt in some water and add half of the kefir whey to it.

4. Pour this brine into the jar until the fish is submerged by it.

5. After that, you tightly close the jar and leave to ferment for 3-5 days at room temperature, then remove and store in the fridge.

6. This can be served with vegetables, spring onion, fresh dill, and some mayonnaise.

Stir Fry Mushroom Leek

Prep time: 15 mins
Cook time: 15 mins
Total time: 30 mins
Serves: 6

Ingredients

3 cups oyster mushrooms (sliced & roots removed)
1 cup sprouted beans
1 onion (thinly sliced)
3 cloves of crushed garlic
1 inch of minced ginger
1 carrot (sliced)
2 leeks (sliced into rings)
1 tsp cumin
5 oz (150g) rice noodles (kindly omit if you are doing GAPS)
½ cup soy (also known as tamari) sauce
½ tsp chili
1 tbsp coconut oil

How You Make It

1. First, boil the rice noodles using the package instructions and set aside in cold water.

2. Next, you heat the coconut oil and add the cumin for 30 seconds till fragrant.

3. Once that is achieved, add onion, garlic, and ginger and then fry for 3 min after which you add the leeks and continue frying until slightly browned.

4. Throw in the mushrooms, sprouted beans and carrot, and stir-fry together till mushrooms become soft before including the soy sauce, chili, and noodles (now cooked).

5. Now, let stir and cook for 2 more minutes, stirring occasionally

6. Serve when done.

Lamb Sausages with Cucumbers

Ingredients

2 large pickled cucumbers
2 organic lamb sausages
1 tsp olive (or coconut oil)

How You Make It

1. Simply rub oil on the sausages so they don't stick to the skillet

2. When done, pan-grill the sausages in the skillet over medium-high heat until well browned

3. Serve with the sliced pickles.

Tahini & Mustard Chicken Spread

Prep time: 10 mins
Total time: 10 mins
Servings: 12

Ingredients

½ chicken (cooked)
2 tbsp of tahini paste
2 tbsp of miso paste
2 tbsp of dijon mustard
2 tbsp of olive oil (or coconut oil)
2 tbsp of truffle oil (optional)

How You Make It

1. First, separate the chicken flesh from the bones and mash them with your hands, removing all smaller bone pieces.

2. Next, combine with the tahini paste, miso, and mustard after which you mash all the ingredients together with your hand until they become smooth.

3. Serve.

Chia Seed Pudding

Prep time: 5 mins
Cook time: 15 mins
Total time: 20 mins
Serves: 2

Ingredients

½ cup of chia seeds
2 cups of coconut milk (or any nut milk)
sea salt to taste
2 handfuls of fresh raspberries
½ tsp vanilla essence
1 tbsp coconut oil or butter (optional)
1 tsp honey

How You Make It

1. First, warm up the milk without bringing to a boil and add a pinch of salt to it.

2. Next, whisk the chia seeds in and add the coconut butter or oil (if using).

3. Let stand for 10 to 15 minutes, then reheat or allow to cool completely.

4. Before serving, whisk in the raspberries and drizzle with honey.

R. Sweet Potato Wedges

Prep time: 10 mins
Cook time: 45 mins
Total time: 55 mins
Serves: 4-6

Ingredients

4 medium-sized sweet potatoes (cut into wedges)
2 tbsp coconut oil (warmed to liquid)
sea salt
pepper and a touch of chili flakes
Ras El Hanout, a Moroccan spice blend (optional)
One or all of (dry tarragon, cumin, oregano or thyme)

How You Make It

1. Begin by preheating your oven to 425F. After which you toss the sweet potatoes with the coconut oil, sea salt, pepper, and herbs.

2. When done tossing, lay them out on a parchment paper and bake for 45 minutes. (be sure to turn from time to time).

Braised Green Cabbage

Prep time: 15 mins
Cook time: 2 hours
Total time: 2 hours 15 mins
Serves: 4

Ingredients

1 medium head of cabbage (cut into wedges)
1 large carrot (chopped)
¼ cup olive oil
1 large yellow onion (cut into thin wedges)
¼ cup chicken stock (or water)
⅛ chili flakes
sea salt

How You Make It

1. First, preheat your oven to 325F.

2. Arrange the cabbage in a baking pan and spread the onion and carrot on top.

3. When done with that, pour the stock into the baking pan and sprinkle with the olive oil, salt, pepper, and chili flakes.

4. Seal the top and bake until the cabbage is very tender (takes about 1.5 hours).

5. When done, take off the cover and bake for additional 15 minutes for the cabbage to get crispy and brown.

Arugula Smoked Fish

Prep time: 7 mins
Total time: 7 mins
Servings: 2

Ingredients

2 handfuls of baby arugula
1 tbsp of balsamic vinegar (or lemon juice)
smoked fish (mackerel or white fish) (make sure it's free of nitrates)
1 avocado
4 tbsp of olive oil
¼ tsp of sea salt

How You Make It

1. Simply combine the arugula with the smoked fish (torn into chunks), and avocado slices in a bowl.

2. Next, whisk the olive oil together with the balsamic vinegar, and salt so they emulsify.

3. Once that's achieved, pour the dressing over arugula.

Veggie & Sausage Delight

Prep time: 15 mins
Cook time: 15 mins
Total time: 30 mins
Servings: 2

Ingredients

½ chopped onion
2 cloves chopped garlic
1 cup chopped asparagus
½ cup sliced carrots
1 cup chopped zucchinis
½ tbsp parsley
1 cup sliced mushrooms
2 tsp coconut oil (or ghee) melted
½ tbsp basil
1 –2 sausages (cooked & chopped)
Sea salt to taste
pepper to taste

How You Make It

1. First, heat the coconut oil and sauté the chopped onions and garlic in it until the onions become soft and translucent.

2. Next, add the rest of the ingredients except the sausages and sauté for 6 to 10 minutes.

3. After that, include the sausages and heat for an additional 5 minutes then serve!

Fish Soup

Prep time: 15 minutes
Cooking time: 4-24 hours
Yield: 3 quarts

Ingredients

3-4 whole fish carcasses (non-oily fish such as sole, rockfish, turbot, or snapper)
2 tbsp butter
1 carrot (chopped)
3 sticks celery (chopped)
2 onions (chopped)
4 cloves garlic
several sprigs of parsley
1-inch ginger (grated)
several sprigs of thyme
1 bay leaf
¼ cup apple cider vinegar
about 3 quarts of water (filtered)

How You Make It

1. First, melt the butter, and cook all the vegetables gently for about 30 minutes until they become soft.

2. Next, add the apple cider vinegar, along with the fish and cover with water.

3. Bring this to a boil and skim off the scum/impurities as they rise to the top.

4. At this point, tie the herb stems together and throw into the pot.

5. Simmer this for 4-24 hours and allow to cool.

6. When cool, you can then strain some of the liquid and use as fish stock.

Coconut Almond Banana Muffins

Prep time: 15 mins
Cook time: 30 mins
Total time: 45 mins
Servings: 6 muffins

Ingredients

2 ripe bananas (mashed)
½ tsp baking powder
2 tbsp shredded coconut
3 tbsp virgin coconut oil (melted)
¼ tsp sea salt
¼ cup coconut flour
2 tbsp chopped almonds

How You Make It

1. Begin by preheating your oven to 350 degrees F.

2. After that, take out a bowl, and combine the bananas with the coconut oil, baking powder, and salt.

3. Next, you mix the coconut flour into the batter from step 2 until there are no lumps.

4. Fold this into the shredded coconut and almonds.

5. Bake until the tops are brown (takes about 30 mins).

Salad Recipes

Zucchini & Anchovy Salad

Ingredients

1 large zucchini (grated)
2 tbsp of olive oil
1 can anchovies (or sardines) (mashed)
⅓ bunch of dill (chopped)
juice of 1 lemon
sea salt

How You Make It

1. First, beat the olive oil, lemon juice, and sea salt together into a nice vinaigrette.

2. Next, combine the zucchini, anchovies, and dill.

3. After that, pour the vinaigrette over the zucchini slices and mix all together.

4. Serve!

Raw Beetroot & Orange Salad

Prep time: 15 mins
Total time: 15 mins
Servings: 4-6

Ingredients

Salad
4 large beets (peeled & grated)
2 oranges (cut into chunks)
cup of pecan nuts (chopped)
¼ cup chopped fresh parsley
1 shallot (peeled & thinly sliced)

Dressing
juice of 1 orange
½ tsp ground cumin
¼ cup unrefined extra virgin olive oil
sea salt to taste
pepper to taste

How You Make It

1. First, you have to prepare the dressing. To do this, simply whisk all its ingredients together and store in a mason jar.

2. Mix the salad ingredients and dress at the table to suit your tastes.

Tahini Miso Dressing

Ingredients

1.5 tbsp tahini paste
1 tbsp miso paste
1 tbsp olive oil
1-inch fresh ginger root
1 tbsp soya sauce
juice of ½ lemon (or apple cider)
water to dilute

How You Make It

1. It's easy. Simply combine all the ingredients and serve!

Prebiotic Creamy Potato Salad

Prep time: 20 mins
Cook time: 45 mins
Total time: 1 hr 5 mins
Serves: 8-10

Ingredients

2 lb red potatoes (quartered)
4 strips of bacon from pasture-raised pigs
2 tbsp Dijon mustard
¼ cup of brine from ferments (or 2 tbsp apple cider vinegar)
1 tbsp sea salt
¾ cup sauerkraut (lacto-fermented, not in vinegar) (chopped)
¼ cup spring onions (chopped)
¾ cup mayo

How You Make It

1. First, preheat your oven to 350F.

2. Next, you boil the potatoes in salted water with skins on for 45 minutes or until they become tender.

3. After that, you bake the bacon strips until nicely browned (about 45 mins).

4. Take out the potatoes and let cool, then cut into ½-inch cubes.

5. When done cutting, combine with all the remaining ingredients and fold them in gently.

6. You can taste and adjust based on your preferences.

Creamy Broccoli Salad

Prep time: 12 mins
Cook time: 7 mins
Total time: 19 mins
Serves: 4

Ingredients

1 bunch of organic broccoli
1 bunch of asparagus
A handful of sprouted beans

Dressing
1.5 tbsp tahini paste
1 tbsp olive oil
1 tbsp soya sauce
1 tbsp miso paste (white miso preferred)
1-inch fresh ginger root
juice of ½ lemon (or apple cider)
water to dilute

How You Make It

1. First, bring water to a boil and put in your steaming basket to help keep the vegetables off the cooker bottom.

2. Next, chop the broccoli and asparagus and throw into the steaming basket.

3. Steam for 5-7 minutes and prepare the dressing by whisking together the tahini, lemon juice, miso, olive oil, and grated ginger

4. You can add water to the dressing to loosen it a bit if it's too thick.

5. Then, if you like the sprouted beans steamed, throw them in about 1- 2 mins before the end of steaming.

6. When the veggies are done, serve them in a bowl and mix in the dressing

7. Toss till well-covered

Seaweed Cucumber Salad

Prep time: 20 mins
Total time: 20 mins
Servings: 2-4

Ingredients

1 handful of wakame seaweed
¼ cup rice vinegar
1 handful of hijiki seaweed
1 tsp honey
1 cucumber (peeled & thinly sliced)
¼ cup coconut aminos
1 tsp sesame oil
1 daikon (radish) (sliced)
sesame seeds

How You Make It

1. Begin by soaking the wakame and hijiki in warm water for at least 10 minutes.

2. When done, strain and make the dressing by whisking the rice vinegar, aminos, coconut honey and sesame oil.

3. Place the cucumber and daikon in a serving bowl and add the seaweed and the sesame oil dressing.

4. Toss well to combine.

Steamed Collard Greens

Prep time: 10 mins
Cook time: 5 mins
Total time: 15 mins
Serves: 2-3

Ingredients

1 bunch of collard greens
1 tbsp of sesame seeds
⅛ cup olive oil
1 lemon, juice off
salt to taste
pepper to taste
Seaweed, like wakame (soaked for at least 10 mins) (optional)

How You Make It

1. First, wash collard greens thoroughly and cut into 1.5-inch ribbons (be sure to cut out the stem).

2. When done, place in a steam basket and steam for 3 to 5 mins.

3. After that, combine the olive oil, lemon juice, salt, and pepper to taste into a dressing.

4. Toast the sesame seeds in a pan and pour the dressing over collard greens.

5. Add the sesame seeds and seaweed.

Sauerkraut Cumin Salad

Prep time: 7 mins
Total time: 7 mins
Serves: 2

Ingredients

1 cup of sauerkraut (you can get this in the fridge section of the store. It should never contain vinegar)
1 tsp of cumin seeds
1 tsp sea salt
1 tbsp olive oil (or flaxseed oil)

How You Make It

1. Preheat a pan over medium-high heat and roast the cumin seeds in it till fragrant.

2. After that, toss sauerkraut, cumin seeds, and oil together in a bowl and serve.

3. You can add more fat/oil to aid digestion.

Roasted B. Tomatoes Over Kale

Prep time: 5 mins
Cook time: 30 mins
Total time: 35 mins
Servings: 4 to 6

Ingredients

1 bunch of kale
1 cup cherry tomatoes (cut in halves)
1 eggplant (chopped)
vinegar dressing

How You Make It

1. First, preheat your oven to 375F. After which you place the eggplant and cherry tomatoes cut side down in a baking tray.

2. Bake for 30 mins or until the tomato skins turn brown.

3. Steam kale for 3 to 5 minutes and put on a plate.

4. Spoon the roasted tomatoes on top and drizzle the vinegar dressing over each salad serving.

Arugula & Baby Tomatoes Mix

Prep time: 10 mins
Total time: 10 mins
Servings: 4 to 6

Ingredients

4 cups of arugula
1 cup cherry tomatoes
1 avocado

How You Make It

1. First, wash the arugula and tomatoes after which you halve the tomatoes and mix them with the arugula.

2. Next, spoon out the avocado to small chunks and add them.

3. Pour in 4 tbsp of vinegar dressing.

Smoothies & Tea

Eggless Mayonnaise

Prep time: 2 hours
Cook time: 15 mins
Total time: 2 hours 15 mins

Ingredients

1 cup organic cashews (soaked for at least 2 hours)
¼ cup water
¼ cup olive oil
1.5 tsp Dijon mustard
1.5 tbsp lemon juice
½ tsp sea salt
paprika, chlorella, curry powder, spirulina (Optional for flavorings)

How You Make It

1. Place all the ingredients in a blender, and blend until silky smooth.

Avocado & Cocoa Smoothie

Serves: 2

Ingredients

1 tbsp ghee (melted)
1 whole avocado
1 large tbsp pumpkin seeds
Pinch of Himalayan sea salt
¼ cup raw cacao powder
Handful of goji berries (soaked for at least 15 min in warm water)
Handful of raw pecan nuts
Pinch of cinnamon
¼ tsp pure vanilla extract
½ tsp fresh lemon juice
Filtered water

How You Make It

1. Simply throw all the ingredients into your blender and blend.

Super Boost Green Basil Smoothie

Prep time: 15 mins
Total time: 15 mins
Serves: 2

Ingredients

1 small zucchini
A handful of basil
A handful of sprouts
1 carrot
zest from ½ lime
¼ tsp sea salt
¼ cup of olive oil
½ tsp ground cumin
A handful of parsley
2 tsp lime juice
2 cloves of garlic
¼ inch ginger root
½ cup of water

How You Make It

1. Add everything into your blender and blend.

Pumpkin Smoothie

Prep time: 10 mins
Total time: 10 mins
Servings: 1-2

Ingredients

1½ cups lukewarm water
½ cup pumpkin puree from BPA-free can (or you can simply steam & scoop out fresh pumpkin)
2 tbsp flax seed
¼ cup pecans
¼ inch fresh ginger root (grated)
1 date, pitted
¼ tsp cinnamon
a handful of dandelion leaves
1 tbsp tahini
1 tbsp coconut butter (preferably Artisana brand)
¼ tsp pure vanilla extract
¼ tsp Camu camu
A pinch of sea salt

How You Make It

1. Add everything in the blender and puree until silky smooth.

Goji Grapefruit Smoothie

Prep time: 2 hrs 7 mins
Total time: 2 hrs 7 mins
Serves: 1

Ingredients

A handful of dry goji berries (presoaked for at least 2 hours)
½ grapefruit
A handful of hemp seeds
A handful of fresh parsley
1 tbsp of milk thistle
1.5 tbsp of ground flax seed (flax seed meal)
Handful of almonds (or pecans or walnut)
1 cup of filtered water

How You Make It

1. Simply combine all the ingredients in a blender and blend until smooth.

Blackberry Power Smoothie

Prep time: 8 mins
Total time: 8 mins
Serves: 1

Ingredients

A handful of organic blackberries
1.5 tbsp of ground flax seed (flax seed meal)
½ tsp camu Camu powder
A handful of almonds, pecans or walnuts
1 tbsp of coconut oil (or ghee)
A handful of hemp seeds
1 tbsp of milk thistle
1 cup of warm water
1 tbsp of pumpkin seeds (optional)
1 tsp raw honey (optional)

How You Make It

1. Simply combine all the ingredients in a blender and blend until smooth.

Improved Homemade Ginger Ale

Ingredients

½ cup fresh ginger root (peeled and grated)
enough filtered water to fill the jar
3-6 tbsp raw honey
¼ cup fresh lime juice
2 tbsp. raw whey
two large pinches of unrefined sea salt

How You Make It

1. It's easy. Simply combine all the ingredients in a glass jar with a lid and shake it up gently to dissolve the honey.

2. Leave at room temperature for one day after which you strain into two Pellegrino bottles with lids.

3. When done, top off each with Pellegrino and store in the refrigerator.

4. You can drink diluted or full-strength as desired.

Root C. Green Smoothie

Ingredients

1 cup mixed baby greens
1 ripe avocado
1 cucumber
1 cup coconut milk
2 large carrots
1 stick of celery
1 bunch of basil leaves (optional)
1 scoop Pea Protein (Use Rootcology's Organic Pea Protein™ formulated)
Sea salt

How You Make It

1. Add everything into your blender and blend until smooth.

Root C. Green Smoothie 2

Ingredients

1 cup mixed baby greens
1 ripe avocado
1 cucumber
1 cup coconut milk
2 large carrots
1 stick of celery
1 bunch of basil leaves (optional)
1 scoop Pea Protein (Use Rootcology's Organic Pea Protein™ formulated)
Sea salt
1 tbsp Camu powder
1 tbsp Cod Liver Oil
1 tbsp Maca root powder
1 tbsp Turmeric powder

How You Make It

1. Add everything into your blender and blend until smooth.

Thyroid Power Smoothie

Ingredients

2-4 tbsp of virgin coconut oil (melted)
½ cup of organic rolled oats
2 tsp of vanilla
Dash salt
4 cups of frozen strawberries (or any frozen fruit of your choice)
3 cups of grass-fed milk, plain kefir (or coconut milk)
2 bananas, fresh or frozen
2 tbsp of green food powder
2 tbsp of raw honey
8 soy-free egg yolks (optional but I advise you use them)

How You Make It

1. First, you blend the entire ingredient except for the fruit until mixed.

2. After that, you add the fruit and then blend until silky and smooth.

Berry Green Smoothie

Ingredients

1 tbsp tyrosine (sunflower seeds or flax seeds)
1 cup greens (kale, or spinach)
½ cup antioxidants (frozen raspberries or blueberries)
1 cup water

How You Make It

1. Add everything into your blender with a little bit of water and blend until smooth.

Thyroid Green Smoothie

Ingredients

1 bunch organic parsley (or organic cilantro)
1 bunch organic greens (we used kale)
2½ - 3 tbsp of coconut oil
5 stalks fresh crisp celery
1 large cucumber
water (Filtered)

How You Make It

1. Simply add everything into your blender and blend until smooth.

Thyroid Booster Smoothie

Ingredients

1 cup full-fat coconut milk
1 tbsp coconut oil
2 Brazil nuts
1 serving Organifi Complete Protein
1 cup mixed greens
1 stick celery
1 tbsp maca powder
½ avocado
1 pinch dulse flakes
1 cup organic frozen berries

How You Make It

1. Blend all ingredients in your blender and enjoy!

Green Tea Smoothie

½ cucumber
1 carrot
1 tsp olive oil
1 cup green tea
A handful of walnuts

How You Make It

1. Blend all ingredients in your blender and enjoy!

Mango Inspired Smoothie

2 leaves kale
1 cup of water
Yogurt
1 banana
½ mango and ½ papaya

How You Make It

1. Blend all ingredients in your blender and enjoy!

Blueberry Choco Delight

Ingredients

½ cup of frozen blueberries
2 celery stalks
1 scoop of raw meal –garden of life- chocolate flavor
1 cup of unsweetened nut milk
1 cup of romaine lettuce
½ tsp of Ceylon Cinnamon
2 tbsp of almond butter

How You Make It

1. Add all ingredients to your blender and blend until smooth.

Pina Colada Smoothie

Ingredients

1 cup of Organic Pineapple
2 celery stalks
1 tbsp of raw, coconut oil (unprocessed & unfiltered)
1 cup of Coconut Milk
1 tbsp of spirulina
1 tbsp of ground flaxseed
½ cup of ice

How You Make It

1. Add all ingredients to your blender, and blend until smooth.

Homemade Cola drink

Prep time: 5 mins
Total time: 5 mins
Serves: 2

Ingredients

4 drops lime essential oil
2 drop lemon essential oil
2 drop nutmeg essential oil
4 tsp vanilla extract
4 drops orange essential oil
2 drop cardamom essential oil
2 drop cinnamon essential oil
4 tsp maple syrup (or honey or liquid stevia)

How You Make It

1. Simply drop all the essential oils into the vanilla extract, and top with the sweetener of choice.

2. Transfer into two glasses of 8 to 10 oz of bubbly water and serve chilled.

Note: Get quality essential oils that can easily be ingested.

Dairy-Free Turmeric Chai Latte

Prep time: 5 mins
Cook time: 15 mins
Total time: 20 mins
Serves: 2

Ingredients

3 cups of water

Masala chai mix
2 tsp rooibos or black tea
2-inch fresh ginger root (sliced)
5 cloves (crushed)
1 large Ceylon cinnamon stick (broken to pieces)
8 cardamom pods (crushed)
1 tsp fennel seed
½ tsp black peppercorns (crushed)

Other ingredients
3 tbsp ghee or coconut butter
¼ tsp vanilla powder (optional)
2 pitted dates
1 tsp turmeric
½ tsp nutmeg powder (optional)

How You Make It

1. First, place the water and the masala chai ingredients in a saucepan and bring water to a boil.

2. Once that is achieved, reduce the heat and simmer for 10-15 minutes after which you strain and transfer to your blender.

3. Add the dates and ghee to the blender as well and blend on high for 1 minute.

4. Include the turmeric powder and blend again for a few seconds after which you pour into a serving glass/glasses.

5. Sprinkle with vanilla powder and nutmeg powder, if using and enjoy!!

Lemon Ginger Tea

Prep time: 5 mins
Cook time: 5 mins
Total time: 10 mins

Ingredients

Fresh ginger root (an inch)
3 tbsp apple cider vinegar (or lemon juice)
1 tbsp honey (raw, organic)

How You Make It

1. First, crush the ginger root in a mortar using a pestle and pour hot water over them.
2. Cover and let it sit for 5 min and then add the lemon and honey.

Conclusion

Congratulation as you have made it to the end of this book containing 50 New Research-Based Recipes To Help Free The Body From Hashimoto's, Graves', Hypothyroidism & Thyroid Related Problems.

If you have followed the recipes outlined in this book and made them as instructed, you should be able to free your self from the thyroid trap within a few weeks.

Once again, congratulation and thank you for reading.

Made in the USA
Lexington, KY
29 December 2017